Renald Blundell

Bones

AF167388

Renald Blundell

Bones

LAP LAMBERT Academic Publishing

Impressum / Imprint

Bibliografische Information der Deutschen Nationalbibliothek: Die Deutsche Nationalbibliothek verzeichnet diese Publikation in der Deutschen Nationalbibliografie; detaillierte bibliografische Daten sind im Internet über http://dnb.d-nb.de abrufbar.
Alle in diesem Buch genannten Marken und Produktnamen unterliegen warenzeichen-, marken- oder patentrechtlichem Schutz bzw. sind Warenzeichen oder eingetragene Warenzeichen der jeweiligen Inhaber. Die Wiedergabe von Marken, Produktnamen, Gebrauchsnamen, Handelsnamen, Warenbezeichnungen u.s.w. in diesem Werk berechtigt auch ohne besondere Kennzeichnung nicht zu der Annahme, dass solche Namen im Sinne der Warenzeichen- und Markenschutzgesetzgebung als frei zu betrachten wären und daher von jedermann benutzt werden dürften.

Bibliographic information published by the Deutsche Nationalbibliothek: The Deutsche Nationalbibliothek lists this publication in the Deutsche Nationalbibliografie; detailed bibliographic data are available in the Internet at http://dnb.d-nb.de.
Any brand names and product names mentioned in this book are subject to trademark, brand or patent protection and are trademarks or registered trademarks of their respective holders. The use of brand names, product names, common names, trade names, product descriptions etc. even without a particular marking in this works is in no way to be construed to mean that such names may be regarded as unrestricted in respect of trademark and brand protection legislation and could thus be used by anyone.

Coverbild / Cover image: www.ingimage.com

Verlag / Publisher:
LAP LAMBERT Academic Publishing
ist ein Imprint der / is a trademark of
AV Akademikerverlag GmbH & Co. KG
Heinrich-Böcking-Str. 6-8, 66121 Saarbrücken, Deutschland / Germany
Email: info@lap-publishing.com

Herstellung: siehe letzte Seite /
Printed at: see last page
ISBN: 978-3-659-42620-9

Bones

Dr. Renald Blundell

2013

Note for the Author

Bone is that part of the skeletal system which caters for structural stability and protection of the internal organs. It is composed mainly of cells and a collagenous extracellular matrix (type 1 collagen) called osteoid which becomes mineralised by the deposition of calcium hydroxyapatite crystals. It is thus not surprising that another main function of bone is to act as a mineral resevoir. In this way bone is used up according to the body's blood calcium levels; when calcium levels are low bone resorption increases and vice versa, so bone is a dynamic material which is constantly being made and broken down. There are various factors that influence bone density, such as age, genetic factors and others all of which mainly influence the stages of bone remodelling.

I would like to thank my colleagues and friends for their contribution mainly: Dr. M. Camilleri and Dr. S. Galea. Last but not least I would like to thanks my kids Kimberley, Dylan and Cayleen for their continuous support and everyday source of motivation. Finally, I would like to dedicate this book to all patients and people that are suffering.

Dr. Renald Blundell B.Sc. (Melit.), M.Phil. (Melit.), Ph.D.(Edin.), MSB (Lond.), C.Biol., EurProBiol., MIBMS, FRSPH(Lond.), CLJ, BMLJ

Contents

The Biology of Bone

Blundell, R.; Camilleri, M.

Introduction

The cells which make up bone are osteoblasts, osteoclasts and osteocytes. Osteocytes are essentially fully differentiated osteoblasts that become entrapped in the osteoid tissue they produce and thereby transform into osteocytes, which make up 90% of all cells in the adult skeleton. Together with the collagenous bone matrix which is made from osteoblasts themselves, bone is formed. (Sommerfeldt, D.W., Rubin, C.T., 2001). The rates of bone formation and bone resorption vary throughout ones life, new bone is added faster than it is broken down during childhood however after the age of 30 bone loss slowly begins to exceed bone formation. When the rate of bone resorption greatly exceeds that of bone formation various disorders of bone can be seen, such as osteoporosis (Haeney, R.P., 1987).

The Morphology of Bone

Calcium and phosphate metabolism is essential for the maintenance of healthy bone since these ions are a major constituent of bone itself. Bone is composed of a tough organic matrix and deposits of calcium salts. Average compact bone is made up of 70% salts and 30% matrix with the latter being greater in newly formed bone. (Guyton, A.C., 2003)

The major salts making up bone are calcium and phosphate. These salts are deposited in bone as an analogue of geologic mineral hydroxyapatite $[Ca_{10}(PO_4)_6(OH)_2]$. This mineral provides mechanical rigidity and load bearing strength to the bone composite (Avioli, L.V., 1998).

Bone matrix is physiologically mineralized and is unique since it is constantly regenerated throughout life as a consequence of bone turnover. The basic building block of the bone matrix network is type I collagen with trace amounts of type III, V, X, and FACIT collagens being present during certain stages of bone formation (Bilezikian, J.P., *et al.* 1996).

Bone matrix is also composed of ground substance made of extra-cellular fluid and proteoglycans mainly hyaluronic acid and chondroiton sulphate.

The organic matrix provides elasticity and flexibility to bone. Its structure will also influence mineralization since it helps control the deposition of calcium salts. (Avioli, L.V., 1998).

Bone matrix contains within it cells called osteocytes that are found embedded deep within bone in osteocytic lacunae. Osteocytes were originally osteoblasts. The bone forming osteoblasts become entrapped within the bone matrix that they produced, which later becomes calcified. The osteoblasts, which are responsible for production of matrix, are found lining the bone surface as clusters of cuboidal cells. In this manner they line the layer of matrix that they produce which is called osteoid tissue before it is calcified. Osteoblasts have been shown to contain receptors for PTH and cytokines.

Osteoclasts are phagocytic cells for bone resorption. These cells are usually found in contact with the calcified bone surface and within a lacuna resulting from its own absorptive activity. Osteoclasts send out projections onto the bone and secrete acids such as citric acid causing dissolution of bone salts. They also release proteolytic enzymes that will digest and dissolve the organic matrix (Roodman, G.D.,1996).

The collagen fibres in the matrix will provide the tensile strength while Ca^{2+} salts provide compressional strength such that the combined properties provide a stable structure. Changes that occur in the biochemistry of bone are important since they influence bone mechanical properties. Thus the consequent size and distribution of mineral crystals in the bone matrix will determine bone strength (Currey, J.D., *et al.* 1996).

The structure of bone is important since it helps us to understand the pathogenesis of the disease. If there are few crystals, then the mechanical strength is compromised, similarly if there are too many crystals or the crystals or the crystals are larger, as in the case for osteoporosis, the bones become brittle. (Paschalis, E.P., *et al.*1997).

Bone Remodelling

Bone remodelling occurs due to a constant process of bone breakdown and bone formation. Osteoclasts are cells that cause bone breakdown or resorption and osteoblasts are cells that cause bone formation. The process of bone remodelling depends on the action of these two types of cells. It occurs at discrete sites within the skeleton and proceeds in an orderly fashion with bone resorption being followed by bone formation.

Remodelling of Cancellous Bone.

Bone remodelling is a series of discrete cellular events organized both in time and space on the bone surface. The steps involved have been well characterized both in healthy bone and in osteoporotic bone. This process is largely mediated by the activity of osteoblasts and osteoclasts and is a prominent feature of endosteal sites.

At any one time, osteoblasts and osteoclasts normally occupy the minority of the bone surface (10-15%), the remainder of which is covered by quiescent lining cells. In this manner the process of bone remodelling occurs in a series of 4 steps.

- **Activation**

Activation refers to the attraction of osteoclasts to a bone surface and is a measure of the rate of bone remodelling. Healthy bone activation occurs every 10 seconds and thus the number of remodelling sites is proportional to the rate of activation.

The first visible step of bone remodelling is the focal attraction of osteoclasts to the quiescent bone surface which is itself not fully mineralised. This surface is made of a thin lamellar membrane which is composed mostly of collagen and thus it is thought that this surface is not degraded by the action of osteoclasts but by lining cells that secrete enzymes like collagenase thus eroding the collagen in this layer. The osteoclasts degrading the bone are attracted to the region before degradation starts and so are present close to the quiescent surface beforehand. Attraction most likely occurs due to fatigue damage to bone itself, coupled by other biochemical signals (Burger, E.H., *et al.* 1984)

The activation of the osteoclasts may occur between integral membrane proteins (integrins) on osteoclast cell membranes with proteins in bone matrix containing RGD (arginine-glycine-asparagine) amino acid sequences such as osteopontin. Various hormones alter the rate of activation; PTH, TH and calcitriol increase the rate of activation and calcitonin and gonadotropic hormones decrease the rate of activation. Local factors such as interleukin-1, 6, 10 and 11 and Tumour necrosis factor (TNF) also stimulate osteoclast activity.

Stimulants such as calcitriol and PTH will mediate their effects by binding to complimentary receptors present on osteoblasts and not osteoclasts in such a way that the effect that these stimulants have on osteoblasts will in turn increase the activity of osteoclasts. Possible effects on osteoblasts are initiation of release of matrix resorbing enzymes such as collagenases to break down bone or else retraction of osteoblasts thus permitting oteoclasts to work on the exposed bone surface. (refer to Fig1-1)

(Miyauchi, A., *et al. 1991).*

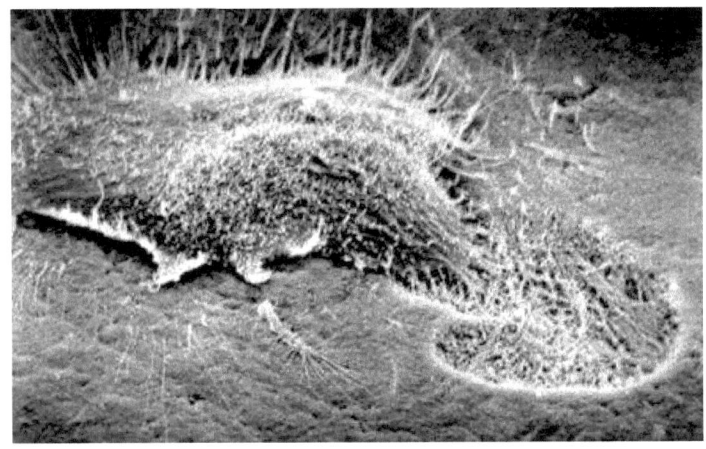

Fig 1-1. Scanning electron micrograph of an osteoclast resorbing bone. (Magnification: ×2000)

(http://www.brsoc.org.uk/gallery/arnett_osteoclast.jpg)

- **Resorption**

The process of resorption first requires the attachment of osteoclasts to bone. This is done so that osteoclasts are intimately related to the underlying bone in such a way that they can mediate their effects more effectively. Following their attachment, osteoclasts can finally initiate the process of bone resorption. This type of bone degradation is brought about by the release of protons and lysosomal enzymes from the ruffled apical borders of these cells that are closely applied to bone. Acid secretion is coupled with release of lysosomal enzymes including β-glucuronidase, carbonic anhydrase and cysteine proteinases like cathepsin- B, which digest collagen under acidic conditions. In this way the bone is literally degraded into various products that make up its various constituents such as the formation of hydroxyproline from the degradation of collagen and the liberation of pyridinoline crosslinks. These degradation products are used as markers for bone resorption and thus may be a useful tool in the identification of osteoporosis.(refer to Fig.1-1) (Baron, R ., *et al.* 1985).

- **Reversal**

Following bone resorption mutinucleated osteoclasts appear to be replaced by mononuclear cells. Over time a layer of cement rich in glycoproteins, acid phosphatase and proteoglycan is formed. This layer is poor in collagen and forms a layer over bone and is responsible for the cessation period between bone resorption and bone formation. In this way the longer the resorption phase, the increased chance of osteoporosis due to no bone formation (Baron, R., *et al.* 1981).

- **Coupling**

Following the formation of the resorption cavity, osteoblasts are attracted to the resorbed surface in a process known as coupling. The coupling signal that attracts osteoblasts is not known. Collagen fragments, bone morphogenic proteins, IGF-II or TGFs appear to act as possible mediators for coupling

(Farley, J.R., *et al.* 1987). In vitro evidence that bone formation many be coupled to resorption by release of mitogen(s) from resorbing bone.

Osteoblasts attach to the bone surface by means of cell surface receptors such as integrins. The infill of new bone depends on the number of osteoblasts that are attracted to the site and the activity of the osteoblasts present, and although the osteoblast activity may be low, if enough osteoblasts are attracted to the site, there will still be adequate bonefill. If coupling has taken place, osteoblasts produce osteoid (collagen and ground substance) at a rate of 0.5-1.0 μm per day.

When the osteoid thickness has reached approximately 12-15 μm, mineralisation begins from the bottom (mineralisation front). At the termination of each remodelling process, the bone surface is again covered by an extremely thin layer of non-mineralised bone and a layer of flat lining cells. The bone is again converted into a resting surface (Mosekilde,L, 1999)

(refer to Fig. 1-2).

The 4 steps making up the remodelling cycle are purposely synchronised in such a way that old bone of inferior quality is continuously replaced by new bone thus it is a mechanism intended to maintain a young skeleton. (refer to Fig 1-2) With each remodelling cycle involving these 4 steps there is a slight deficit in bone formation, such that the total bone loss is therefore a function of the number of cycles in process at any one time. In this manner any factors causing an increased in the rate of activation of bone remodelling will thus increase the proportion of bone remodelling units at any one time and increase bone loss (Kleerekoper, M., *et al.* 1996).

The balance in adults is normally negative (i.e. after each remodelling process there is therefore a reduced mass). There is thus an unavoidable loss of bone mass with age. It also has another cost: it causes disruption of the trabecular network with age. Because the balance is negative, there is a thinning of the trabecular structures in the network (refer to Fig. 1-3), and this makes osteoclastic perforations possible. As the normal resorption depth is approximately 40-50 μm, one resorption site covering more than half of the circumference of a trabecula, or two resorption sites, one on each side of a trabecula, could easily perforate a trabecular structure with a diameter of 90-100 μm [90-120 μm is the normal thickness of horizontal trabeculae in the vertebral body of elderly individuals (refer to Fig. 1-4)].

This increased rate of activation of the remodelling cycle brought about by certain factors is responsible for many cases of secondary osteoporosis, however the loss of bone occurring with aging as in senile osteoporosis appears to result from an imbalance between resorption and formation resulting from impairment of appropriate signalling. This causes inefficient osteoblast recruitment. In this way bone loss does not necessarily occur when there is an increased rate of bone activation but also when the rate of activation decreases.

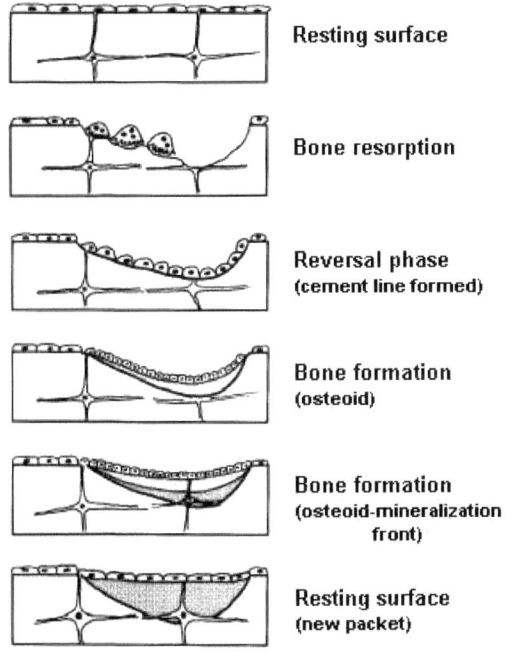

Resting surface

Bone resorption

Reversal phase
(cement line formed)

Bone formation
(osteoid)

Bone formation
(osteoid-mineralization
front)

Resting surface
(new packet)

Fig 1-2: Stages in the remodelling cycle (Mosekilde,L., 1999)

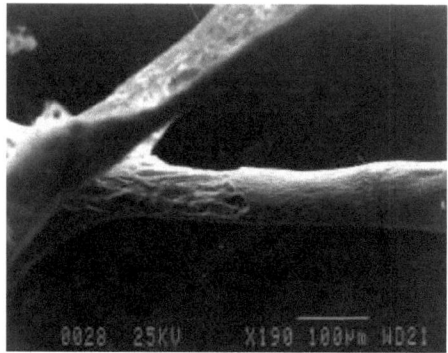

Figure 1-3: Remodelling site on a trabecula shown by use of Scanning Electron Microscopy by use of SEM (Magnification: ×190) (Mosekilde,L., 1999)

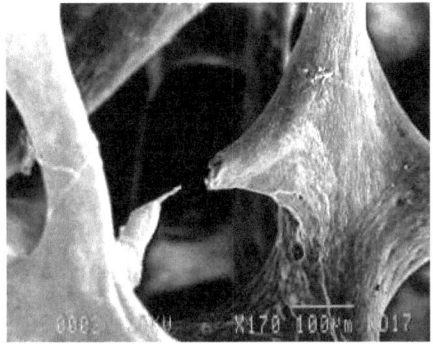

Figure 1-4: Osteoclastic perforation of a thin horizontal trabecula by use of SEM (Magnification: ×170) (Mosekilde,L., 1999)

References

- Avioli LV, Krane SM. Metabolic Bone Disease and Clinically Related Disorders. 3rd ed. San Diego, 1998:23-51.

- Baron, R ., Neff, L., Louvard,D. and Courtuy, P.J. (1985) Cell mediated extracellular acidification and bone resorption: evidence for a low pH in resorbing lacunae and localisation of a hundred small KD lysosomal membrane proteins at the osteoclasts ruffled border. J Cell Biology, 101,2210 - 2222.

- Baron ,R., Vignery, A. and Lang, R. (1981) reversal phase and osteopenia: defective coupling of resorption to formation in the pathogenesis of osteoporosis.

- Bilezikian JP,Raisz LG, Rodan GA,eds. Principles of bone biology.1996:87-102

- Burger,E.H., van der Meer, J.W.N. & Nijweide, P.J. 1984 Osteoclast formation from mononuclear phagocytes: role of bone forming cells. J cell bio, 99, 1901-1906

- Currey JD, Brean K, Zioupos P. The effects of ageing and changes in mineral content in degrading the toughness of human femora. Journal of Biomechanics 1996;29:257-260.

- Farley JR, Tarbauz N, Murphy LA, Masuada T, and Baylink DJ. (1987)

- Guyton, A.C., and Hall, J.E., Endocrinology and Reproduction. 2003;79:987-994

- Haeney RP: Qualitative factors in osteoporotic fracture: The satate of the question. Osteoporosis 1987; (1) : 281

- Kleerekoper M.MD,Avioli LV.MD.,F.A.C.E.1996 Primer on the metabolic diseases chap 94 pp264-271

- Miyauchi A, Alvarez J, Greenfield EM, et al. Recognition of osteopontin and related peptides by an α v β 3 integrin stinulates immediate cell signals in osteoclasts. Journal of Biological Chemistry 1991;266:20369-20374

- Mosekilde L, Eriksen EF, Charles P. Effects of thyroid hormone on bone and mineral metabolism. Endocrinology and metabolism clinics of North America 1990; 19:3563

- Paschalis EP, Betts F, Picarlo E, Mendelsohn R, Boskey AL. Fmicrospectroscopic analysis of human iliac crest biopsies from untreated osteoporotic bone. Calcified Tissue International 1997;61:487-492.

- Roodman GD. Advances in bone biology:the osteoclast. Endocrine Reviews 1996; 17:308-332.

- Sommerfeldt D.W., Rubin C.T.. Biology of bone and how it orchestrates the form and function of the skeleton. European Spine Journal 2001; 10:86-95.

- www.brsoc.org.uk/gallery/arnett_osteoclast.jpg

Physiology of Vitamin D

Blundell, R; Galea, S.

Abstract

Vitamin D is relevant to several processes in the body, mainly in the intracellular mechanisms affecting Parathyroid hormone and calcitonin regulation, regulation of vitamin D production by negative feedback and calcium and phosphorous level regulation. Vitamin D may be synthesised in the dermal layer of the skin or absorbed through the diet and utilised. Its biosynthesis initiates from cholesterol and its derivatives and is followed by a cascade of reactions, completed in the kidneys and transported via the blood to where it is utilized. The vitamin D receptor determines the physiological effects of vitamin D and any mutations will cause imbalances in bone homeostasis.

Keywords: Dihydrocholecalciferol, vitamin D receptor, calcium, parathyroid hormone, phosphate, calcitonin.

Introduction

Vitamin D is mainly synthesised by the skin when exposed to ultraviolet rays. It can also be obtained through the diet as it is found in oily fish, eggs and fortified cow's milk. The active form of vitamin D binds to vitamin D receptors (VDRs) receptors located in bone, the intestines, kidneys, parathyroids and also haematopoietic tissue, cells of the immune system, the prostate in males and several other locations in the body, where it helps normal function to occur (De Luca H.F. and Cantorna M.T., 2004). Ligand binding to the VDR causes heterodimerisation in conjunction with the retinoic X

18

receptor in the nucleus to occur, leading to binding of the heterodimer to Vitamin D response elements (Costanzo L.S, 2006). This vitamin D receptor complex transcriptionally activates genes, including calcium binding genes. The actions of these transcribed genes cause absorption of calcium and phosphate ions. Vitamin D increases calcium entry into cells, movement of calcium through cytoplasm, and transfer of calcium into the circulation. Serum calcium levels are regulated by combined action of vitamin D and parathyroid hormone (Bronner F. and Pansu D., 1999).

1.1 Biosynthesis

Biosynthesis of vitamin D occurs in a series of steps starting from cholesterol being oxidised to provitamin D. Provitamin D is converted to 7-hydrochlesterol by UV light, followed by conversion to pre-vitamin D. This is converted by reversible thermal conversion to vitamin D3 in the skin, which is also known as cholecalciferol. Mechanisms are present to prevent overproduction of vitamin D3 during overexposure to sunlight since excess vitamin D3 is converted to inactive compounds. Vitamin D binding protein (VDBP) takes up vitamin D3 in the blood to the liver, where it is converted to 25-hydroxycholecalciferol (25-$(OH)D_3$). This is taken up by the blood and reaches the kidneys, where it is converted to 1,25-dihydroxycholecalciferol (1,25-$(OH)_2D_3$); the active metabolite of vitamin D, and 24,25-dihydroxycholecalciferol; which is inactive (Costanzo L.S., 2006). Vitamin D2 originating from ergosterol in plants, a dietary supplement is metabolised in a similar way (Passieri G. *et al.*, 2008).

1.1.1 Transcriptional regulation of Vitamin D_3

The levels of 25-$(OH)D_3$ are regulated by a negative feedback response, which inhibits its production from vitamin D3. This is important since the converted form of vitamin D is not stored and has a half-life of two weeks, as opposed to the vitamin D3 form which can be stored in the liver for months. Parathyroid hormone (PTH) controls the production of $1,25-(OH)_2D_3$ in the proximal convoluted tubules. The conversion of $25-(OH)D_3$ to $1,25-(OH)_2D_3$ is almost entirely dependent upon PTH. Calcium itself inhibits the formation of $1,25-(OH)_2D_3$ and since it suppresses PTH secretion, calcium also causes indirect inhibition of the active metabolite formation. In higher plasma concentrations, calcium also promotes formation of inactive 24,25-dihydroxycholecalciferol, which is useful since less Ca uptake from bone, the small intestine and distal renal tubules occurs, bringing serum Ca back to normal levels, around 9.4mg/dL (Guyton A.C. and Hall J.E., 2005).

Figure 1.1: A diagram showing sources of vitamin D in the diet and the main processes of vitamin D synthesis, metabolism and its effects on the intestine and bone.

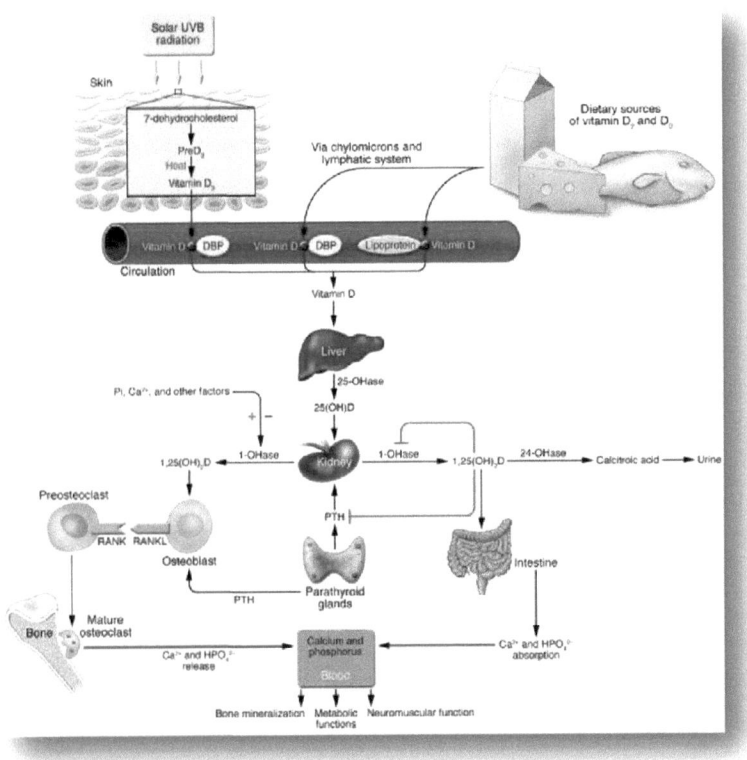

The red lines indicate feedback inhibition of Parathyroid Hormone and 1α-hydroxylase, whilst the green positive sign and red negative sign show enhancement and inhibition of 1α-hydroxylase. Receptor activator for nuclear kB (RANK) stimulates osteoclastic activity in bone (http://www.jci.org/articles/view/29449/figure/3).

1.1.2 Actions of Vitamin D

The actions of vitamin D in its active hormone form are various and more of its importance in the body is being discovered, such as in the reproductive; especially prostate metabolism, and immune system. Its functions related to bone homeostasis are the following; intestinal calcium and phosphate absorption and decreased calcium and phosphate excretion by the kidneys. $1,25-(OH)_2D_3$ increases calcium binding protein, calbindins and calcium channel TRPV6 production in the enterocytes, which functions as a transporter for calcium across the cells and into the bloodstream. This protein is stored within cells even if $1,25-(OH)_2D_3$ is excreted and so calcium uptake continues. $1,25-(OH)_2D_3$ also stimulates the formation of a calcium-stimulated ATPase as well as alkaline phosphatase, which seem to promote calcium uptake. When vitamin D is present in great quantities, it causes absorption of bone by activating osteoblasts which in turn activate osteoclast action. However, in smaller quantities vitamin D causes bone calcification, since it increases bone mineralisation by modulating calcium influx and increasing calcium binding proteins; such as osteocalcin and osteoportin, in osteoblasts (Bouillon R. *et al.*, 2008).

2.1 The Vitamin D Receptor (VDR)

2.1.1.1 VDR expression and its actions in bone

VDR is a receptor expressed by almost all cells in the body and belongs to the steroid receptor family. VDR functions by heterodimerisation together with any of the three isomers for retinoid X receptor (RXR) lacking the specific ligand 9-cis-retinoic acid. When $1,25-(OH)_2D_3$ binds to this complex, the active ligand binding domain (LBD) is formed and this complex diffuses through the cell membrane, as $1,25-(OH)_2D_3$ is a lipid soluble hormone. Once this receptor is activated, a cascade of reactions occur including activation of the MAP-kinase (mitogen activated protein kinase) pathway and an intracellular increase in cyclic adenosine monophosphate (cAMP), protein kinase C (PKC) and opening of calcium and chloride channels, resulting in a biological response. The main pathway for activation, however, is through vitamin D response element (VDRE) activation by binding of the LBD of the VDR to a specific region, where zinc fingers seem to play a role of aiding this binding. This modulates gene expression in the nucleus and depending on the cell where it is active, different actions will be brought about. For instance, in osteoblasts calcium and chloride channels open; which are essential for bone mineralisation and the production of the plasma membrane protein receptor activator of NF-κB ligand (RANKL), which promotes osteoclast development. Furthermore, in intestinal cells transcaltachia (rapid transport of calcium), and activation of MAP-kinase, PKC, and phospholipase C occurs (Norman A.W., 2008).

2.1.2 Polymorphisms of the VDR

A study by Bouillon R. *et al.,* was carried out to see the effects of mutations or loss of VDRs in mice. It was found that these mice were suffering from severe hypocalcemia, osteomalacia and rickets, as a result of imbalance in calcium and bone homeostasis; due to $1,25\text{-}(OH)_2D_3$ (calcitriol) not being able to act on the receptors. Also, phosphate and PTH balance, intestinal absorption and renal calcium reabsorption, seem to be processes dependent on calcitriol activated genes because the mice showed signs of hypophophatemia, secondary hyperparathyroidism, requirement of activation of genes coding for TRPV6, CaBP-9k, $PMCA_{10}$ in the intestine and TRPV5 in renal tubular epithelium. These transporters mentioned above; with the exception of TRPV5, do not seem to be entirely dependent on activation by the VDRE complex since the mice did not develop a significant decrease in calcium absorption. This could be due to the presence of other receptors in the enterocytes responsible for calcium uptake.

Figure 1.2: Vitamin D_3 synthesis and its transport to target cells

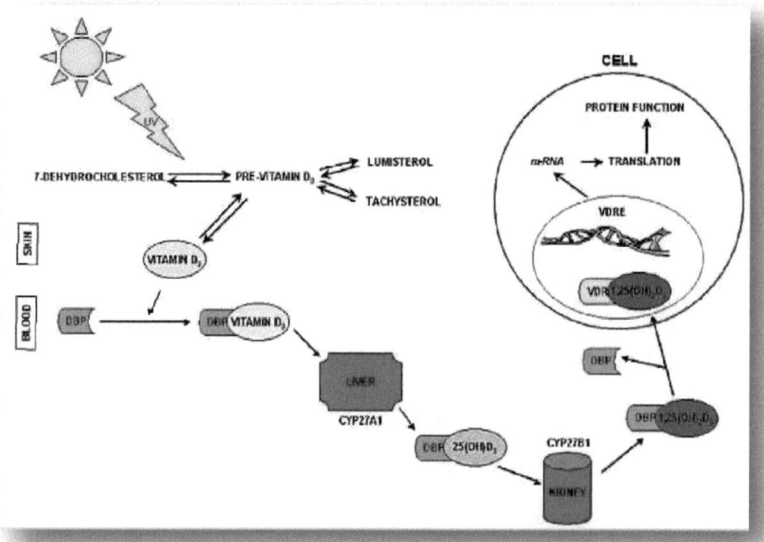

This diagram shows the pathway taken from synthesis of vitamin D in the skin (forming inactive metabolites lumisterol and tachysterol when exposed to excess UV rays) to binding to vitamin D binding protein (DBP) and metabolism by cytochrome P450 oxidase in the liver (encoded by the gene CYP27A1). DBP carries 25-(OH)D_3 to the kidneys, where another cytochrome P450 oxidase; this time encoded by CYP27B1 in the proximal tubules of the kidneys, produces 1,25-(OH)$_2D_3$. This dissociates from DBP once it reaches the target cell and binds to vitamin D receptor (VDR). Within the nucleus, binding to the vitamin D response element (VDRE) induces translation of genes to synthesise proteins needed for a particular function.

(http://www.bioscience.org/2001/v6/d/hansen/figures.htm)

24

Figure 1.3: VDR ligand binding and its intracellular cascade of reactions

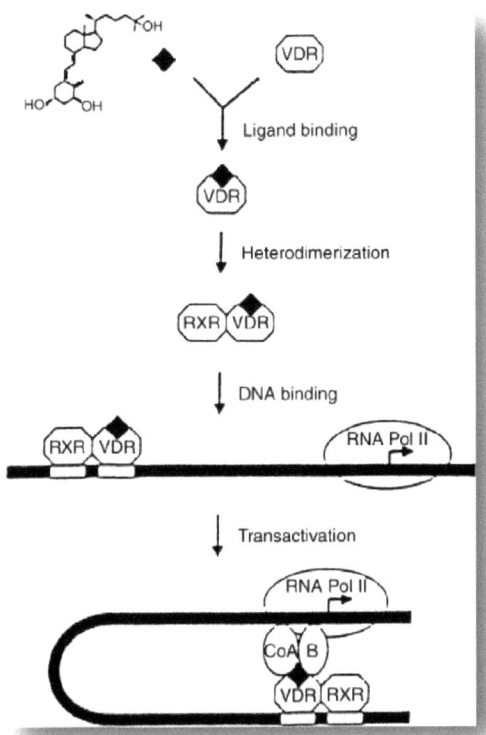

Binding of 1,25-dihydroxycholecalciferol causes heterodimerization with retinoid X receptor to occur. This complex binds to DNA and after transactivation has occurred, it binds to RNA polymerase 2, as well as coenzyme A (Co A) and transcriptional factor IIB (denoted here as B). (http://www.nature.com/ki/journal/v56/n73s/fig_tab/4491279f1.html)

Conclusion

In conclusion the actions of vitamin D in the body are vast and anything causing an imbalance in this hormone results in consequences such as rickets, osteoporosis and promotion of cancer growth. A decrease in vitamin D levels may be due to several reasons including polymorphisms of the VDR as well as mutations in the enzymes involved in its biosynthesis. Vitamin D is involved in calcium and phosphate absorption and so these are essential to bone growth and functions. Its interaction with parathyroid hormone and calcitonin is evident; consequently allowing tight regulation of calcium and phosphate levels, ensuring that homeostasis within the body is maintained.

References

1. Bouillon R., Carmeliet G., Verlinden L., Van Etten E., Verstuyf A., Luderer H.F., Lieben L., Mathieu C. and Demay M. (2008). Vitamin D and Human Health: Lessons from Vitamin D Receptor Null Mice. *Endocr. Rev.* 2008; **29(6)**: 726–776.

2. Bronner F. and Pansu D. (1999). Nutritional aspects of Calcium absorption. *J. Nutr.* 1999 January; **129(l)**: 98-108.

3. Costanzo L.S. (2006). Physiology (3rd ed.). Elsevier, Philadelphia, U.S.A. (ISBN: 978-1-4160-2320-3)

4. De Luca H.F. and Cantorna M.T. (2001). Vitamin D: Its role and uses in immunology. *FASEB J.* 2001 December; **80 (6 suppl):** 1689S-1696S.

5. Guyton A.C., Hall J.E. (2005). Textbook of Medical Physiology (11th ed.). Elsevier, Philadelphia, U.S.A. (ISBN-13: 978-0-7216-0240-0)

6. Norman A.W. (2008). $1\alpha,25(OH)_2$ Vitamin D_3 Vitamin D Nuclear Receptor (VDR) and Plasma Vitamin D-Binding Protein (DBP) Structures and Ligand Shape Preferences for Genomic and Rapid Biological Responses. In: Bilezikian J.P., Raisz L.G. and Martin T.J. (Eds.). *Principles of Bone Biology*, Volume 1 (3rd ed.) (pp. 750-764) Academic Press Inc., New York. U.S.A. (ISBN-13: 978-0123738844)

7. Passeri G., Vescovini R., Sansoni P., Galli C., Franceschi C., Passeri M., and The Italian Multicentric Study on Centenarians (IMUSCE) (2008). Calcium metabolism and vitamin D in the extreme longevity. *Exp. Gerontol.* 2008 February; **43(2)**: 79–87.

Websites

- http://www.bioscience.org/2001/v6/d/hansen/figures.htm
- http://www.jci.org/articles/view/29449/figure/3
- http://www.nature.com/ki/journal/v56/n73s/fig_tab/4491279f1.html

Parathyroid Hormone and Calcitonin regulating Calcium levels

Blundell, R.; Galea, S.

Abstract

Maintaining normal calcium levels within the body (8.5-10mg/dL) requires the action of two hormones in particular; parathyroid hormone (PTH) and calcitonin (http://www.bloodbook.com/ranges.html). In lower calcium levels, PTH is released and works in such a way as to increase the calcium back to the normal range. Calcitonin acts exactly in the inverse way by targeting osteoclasts and osteoblasts. A somewhat constant amount of calcium is lost from the body through fecal excretion. In the gut, absorption and secretion of calcium and phosphate occurs, depending on the free ionized calcium in the extracellular fluid. The amount of calcium in the extracellular fluid also influences excretion of calcium in the renal system. The largest pool of calcium is found in bone, which is essential in calcium homeostasis. This is because through bone remodelling, calcium may be taken up from the extracellular fluid or given up to the extracellular fluid depending on the presence of hormones in a process known as osteolytic osteolysis. The processes mentioned above are mediated through PTH, calcitonin and 1,25-dihydroxycholecalciferol.

Keywords: Calcium, parathyroid hormone, calcitonin, bone, vitamin D and phosphate.

Introduction

Calcium has several important functions in the body, including enzymatic regulation (e.g. calmodulin), neuromuscular function, blood coagulation and hormone secretion. The free ionized calcium levels making up 48% of calcium in the blood, fluctuates and hormones act on this form on calcium to restore homeostasis. 99% of calcium in the

28

body is found in the form of hydroxyapatite crystals which make up the inorganic component of bone. Trabecular bone is important to calcium turnover in bone, as it presents with a greater surface area and so it is highly accessible. Bone mineralisation and resorption are regulated by PTH and vitamin D, in contrast to calcitonin which stimulates bone formation only (Blair H.C *et al*, 2007).

1. Parathyroid Hormone actions and Calcium regulation

PTH, secreted by chief cells in the parathyroid glands, is essential in regulating calcium and phosphate levels in the body by influencing intestinal absorption, renal excretion as well as ion exchange between the extracellular fluid and bone fluid across the osteocytic membrane. Maximal PTH secretion occurs at calcium levels below 3.5mg/dL and is inhibited at levels above 5.5mg/dL. In low calcium levels, adenylyl cyclase is activated, causing an increase in intracellular cyclic AMP. Phospholipase C is inhibited, causing a decrease in inositol triphosphate and in turn, a decrease in intracellular calcium. These processes stimulate high levels of PTH secretion.

PTH causes bone absorption of calcium and phosphate from bone by two ways; activating osteocytes and osteoblasts within minutes to hours and stimulating haematopoeitic tissue for osteoclast proliferation. After a few days, secondary signals activate the fully matured osteoclasts to increase reabsorption of bone itself and not selectively taking up calcium and phosphate ions from the bone reservoir. Absorption of salts takes place readily; since they are extremely small and have a high surface area exposed to extracellular fluid and blood (about 5% of the cardiac output is distributed to bone). PTH promotes the formation of vitamin D_3 in the kidneys and therefore indirectly promotes calcium absorption through the gut. PTH prevents calcium excretion in the distal convoluted tubules in the kidneys by stimulating its reabsorption, whose actions are mediated via the PTH receptor. Mutations in the PTH receptor cause problems such as hypocalcemia and Jansen's metaphyseal chondrodysplasia amongst others, showing how important PTH intracellular

29

mechanisms are to calcium homeostasis. PTH also increases inorganic phosphate elimination by the kidneys by inhibiting its reabsorption in the distal tubules of the kidneys (Pettway G.J. *et al*, 2007).

Continued PTH stimulation for months results in weakened bones, thus osteoblasts are activated simultaneously in an attempt to mineralise bone. Since bone is a buffer-reservoir of calcium and contains about 1000 times as much calcium as the extracellular fluid, the effect of weakened bones is not immediately observed. However, in severe calcium deficiency or prolonged PTH secretion; commonly caused by vitamin D deficiency in children and the elderly, leading to secondary hyperparathyroidism, bone cavities containing multinucleated osteoclasts can be found after several months. The mitochondria of tissues, such as the intestines, are rich in calcium and also aid the buffering system as exchange across to the extracellular fluid occurs to maintain constant calcium levels (Pettway G.J. *et al.*, 2008).

1.1   Idiopathic Hypercalciuria and Calcium sensing receptors

In a study by Worcester E.M. and Coe F.L. (2009), it was found that increased calcium bone loss results in idiopathic hypercalciuria (IH), which in turn causes kidney stones. Usually, in bones which are no longer growing in healthy non-pregnant adults, calcium absorption is matched by renal excretion. This is sufficient for the maintenance of bone unless there is a pathological reason for excess excretion (i.e. >250mg/day in females and >300mg/day in males in urine). IH was found to be a complex polygenic trait which is largely dependent on the diet. It was found that a low calcium diet results in a negative calcium balance, despite increased intestinal uptake and decreased renal excretion in IH. The continual loss of calcium from resorption is a detriment to the skeletal system and growth. This condition also causes an increase in VDR receptors, however, there is no significant increase in $1,25\text{-}(OH)_2D_3$ which could point to increased effectiveness of $1,25\text{-}(OH)_2D_3$ due to increased receptors. Calcium sensing receptors (CaSR) responsive to 1,25-$(OH)_2D_3$ and located in parathyroid, renal, bone and intestinal tissues in these patients, were found to be mutated having a gain in function. This abnormality along with VDR polymorphisms is considered to be a contributing factor to the disease. PTH levels in these patients were normal or slightly low; however, PTH seems to be suppressed therefore causing less calcium reabsorption from the late distal and collecting tubules.

1.2   Intracellular PTH mediated mechanisms

Cyclic AMP seems to mediate most of PTH's effects by a secondary messenger mechanism, since it increases rapidly in its effecter cells including osteocytes and osteoclasts. Osteoclastic secretion of enzymes and acids which cause bone resorption and formation of 1,25-$(OH)_2D_3$ may be dependent on cAMP mechanisms. A slight decrease in calcium detected by the CaSRs in the parathyroid glands causes an immediate increase in secretion of PTH and the opposite occurs in an increase in calcium serum concentration (Guyton A.C. and Hall J.E., 2005). Osteoclasts also possess a calcium sensing function; when a fluctuation of as much as 8-20mM is detected, hydroxyapatite dissolution occurs by stimulated osteoclasts. The ryanodine receptor molecule (RyR) seems to aid osteoclast regulation when it comes to calcium influx and efflux and possibly calcium sensing, however, its role remains unclear (Blair H.C. *et al.*, 2007).

1.3   OPG/RANK/RANK-L system and bone remodelling

A protein belonging to the Tumour Necrosis Factor superfamily, RANK-L (receptor activator nuclear factor kB ligand), its receptor RANK (receptor activator nuclear factor kB) and osteoprotegerin (OPG) seem to play a key role in bone resorption. RANK is a receptor found on osteoclasts, RANK-L is transcribed by osteoblasts, bone marrow stromal cells and T-lymphocytes and OPG is expressed on osteoblasts. PTH and vitamin

D seem to be involved in OPG and RANK-L regulation and expression on cells, consequently regulating bone remodelling. Remodelling occurs in steps including activation, resorption, reversal and formation. Although OPG numbers increase in people above 70 years of age, the OPG/RANK/RANK-L mechanisms involved in preventing bone loss deem to be insufficient. PTH in the elderly is increased resulting in increased calcium in the extra- and intra-cellular fluid. However, these patients are usually suffering from vitamin D hypovitaminosis; due to a reduction in amount of 7-dehydrocholesterol in the skin required for vitamin D synthesis, as well as more time spent indoors with insufficient exposure to UV light and low vitamin D (and calcium) intake in the diet (Kearns A.E., Khosla S. and Kostenuik P.J., 2008).

2. Calcitonin regulating calcium and phosphate levels

Calcitonin has the opposite effects of PTH as it depresses calcium concentration in the extracellular fluid. It is secreted by the parafollicular cells (C cells) in the follicles of the thyroid gland in response to increased calcium levels. Therefore, it inhibits the absorptive action of osteoclasts, as well as osteolytic activities and amorphous calcium phosphate exchange across the osteocytic membrane. Consequently, it deposits excess calcium in the form of calcium salts. A long term effect of calcitonin is to decrease osteoclast formation resulting in decreased osteoblast numbers and it exchanges calcium despite laying down mineral salts on the bone matrix. However, calcitonin has a limited effect on calcium homeostasis, since studies have shown that following a thyroidectomy, the calcium ion concentration is not significantly changed. The rates of absorption and deposition are very low in humans, thus decreased absorption due to calcitonin does not impact extracellular calcium concentration unless a pathological condition is present; such as Paget's disease, in which osteoclasts are highly activated. Also, as calcitonin increases, PTH decreases and vice versa (Davey R.A. *et al.*, 2008).

Conclusion

Both PTH and calcitonin work in influencing calcium and phosphate levels and are released depending on the activation of the calcium sensitive cells. These hormones affect each other as well as vitamin D and maintain calcium within a narrow range. A loss of control in calcium levels is detrimental, as can be seen in conditions such as idiopathic hypercalciuria, primary hyperparathyroidism, pseudohypoparathyroidism, hypercalcemia due to malignancy and Jansen's metaphyseal chondrodysplasia; where a PTH receptor defect is involved.

References

8. Blair H.C., Schlesinger P.H., Huang C.L.H. and Zaidi M. (2007). Calcium signalling and calcium transport in bone disease. *Biochem*. 2007; **45**: 539–562.

9. Davey R.A, Turner A.G, McManus J.F, Chiu WS. M., Tjahyono F., Moore A.J, Atkins G.J, Anderson P.H., Ma C., Glatt V., MacLean H.E, Vincent C., Bouxsein M., Morris H.A., Findlay D.M. and Zajac J.D. (2008). Calcitonin Receptor Plays a Physiological Role to Protect Against Hypercalcemia in Mice. *J. Bone Miner. Res*. 2008 August; **23(8)**: 1182–1193.

10. Guyton A.C., Hall J.E. (2005). Textbook of Medical Physiology (11th ed.). Elsevier, Philadelphia, U.S.A. (ISBN-13: 978-0-7216-0240-0)

11. Kearns A.E., Khosla S. and Kostenuik P.J. (2008). Receptor Activator of Nuclear Factor κB Ligand and Osteoprotegerin Regulation of Bone Remodeling in Health and Disease. *Endocr. Rev*. **29(2)**: 155–192.

12. Pettway G.J., Meganck J.A., Koh A.J, Keller E.T, Goldstein S.A and McCauley L.K. (2007) Parathyroid Hormone Mediates Bone Growth through the Regulation of Osteoblast Proliferation and Differentiation. *Bone*. 2008 April; **42(4)**: 806–818.

13. Worcester E.M. and Coe F.L. (2008). New Insights into the Pathogenesis of Idiopathic Hypercalciuria. *Semin. Nephrol*. 2008 March; **28(2)**: 120–132.

Websites

-   http://www.bloodbook.com/ranges.html
-   http://www.jci.org/articles/view/29449/figure/3

Clinical Correlates Involving Deficiency of Vitamin D and Calcium

Blundell, R.; Galea, S.

Abstract

The effects of vitamin D and calcium deficiency are evident in several patients suffering from various diseases, including osteoporosis and rickets. Other hormones, such as glucocorticoids, also play a role in bone homeostasis leading to bone growth promotion or retardation. Consequently, hormone imbalances in patients should be considered with suspected vitamin D and calcium deficiency.

The deficiency of vitamin D and calcium lead to non-bone related abnormalities, for instance promotion of prostate cancer and retardation of blood clotting respectively. However, this article will be focusing on the detrimental effects of osteoporosis and rickets on patients. Vitamin D and calcium deficiency may be prevented by adequate sun exposure as well as diet supplementation. Vitamin D and calcium deficiency result in lack of intracellular mechanisms, loss of bone matrix and density, hence weaker bones. This leads to an increased probability of bone fractures (Dowd and Stafford, 2008).

Keywords: Vitamin D, calcium, osteoporosis, rickets, diet, deficiency.

Introduction

Several diseases such as osteoporosis, rickets, osteomalacia and rheumatoid arthritis have been linked with problems due to bone metabolism, often involving deficiency of vitamin D and calcium. The recommended daily dietary intake of vitamin D is 600IU, ideally increased to 800IU in the elderly, apart from having adequate exposure to UV light (http://ods.od.nih.gov/factsheets/vitamind). Vitamin D rich foods include oily fish, milk and eggs as mentioned previously. Calcium rich sources include milk, cheese and yoghurt and the recommended daily intake is summarized in the table below. According to Dowd and Stafford in *The Vitamin D Cure* (2008), ideal vitamin D levels should be between 50 and 70, and additional calcium supplementation is unnecessary if the diet is acid-base balanced. For instance, in osteoarthritis, the disease in bone remodelling occurs due to vitamin deficiency and acid excess in the diet. Therefore, calcium supplementation would be unlikely to improve the prognosis of the patient.

Calcium is absorbed in the small intestine via proteins such as TRPV6, calbindin 9K, PMCA1, and NCX1 and a small percentage remains in the intestines to be egested in the stools. Since vitamin D is lipid soluble, when obtained through the diet it diffuses through intestinal epithelium. Until recently, it was thought that people suffering from Crohn's disease and coeliac disease have impaired calcium and vitamin D uptake (Douard V. *et al.*, 2010). This would increase the risks having of bone fractures, rickets in growing children and osteoporosis. However, in a study shown by Kumari M. *et al.* (2010), it was found that young men having stable Crohn's disease do not have impaired calcium uptake. It was only in patients who had inflammatory Crohn's disease that calcium uptake was impaired and this problem was solved by administering vitamin D as it has been suggested to increase calcium transporting proteins and decrease the inflammatory response. This treatment was also found to reduce bone turnover markers and TNF-α levels.

1.1 The role of other hormones in maintaining bone homeostasis

Disorders in growth hormone (GH), glucocorticoids, insulin-like growth factors (IGFs), thyroid hormones and steroids (such as oestrogens) also affect bone growth. For instance, glucocorticoids given to children may stunt bone growth. Receptors for glucocorticoids are found on osteoblasts and so it seems to be important in bone formation and mineral deposition. However, it was discovered that when given to mice in pharmacological doses chronically, apoptosis of osteoblasts and osteocytes and inhibition of osteoblast proliferation occurs, resulting in osteoporosis (Karaplis A.C., 2008).

Table 4: A table showing the recommended daily amount of calcium in the diet.

Age	Male	Female	Pregnant	Lactating
0–6 months*	200 mg	200 mg		
7–12 months*	260 mg	260 mg		
1–3 years	700 mg	700 mg		
4–8 years	1,000 mg	1,000 mg		
9–13 years	1,300 mg	1,300 mg		
14–18 years	1,300 mg	1,300 mg	1,300 mg	1,300 mg
19–50 years	1,000 mg	1,000 mg	1,000 mg	1,000 mg
51–70 years	1,000 mg	1,200 mg		
71+ years	1,200 mg	1,200 mg		

* Adequate Intake (AI)

The table above shows that there is the highest requirement for calcium intake from 9-18 years of age. Pregnant and lactating females do not seem to require a higher calcium intake than that which is considered normal for their age group. Post-menopausal females need a higher calcium intake than males due to their higher risk of developing osteoporosis.

(http://ods.od.nih.gov/factsheets/calcium)

Figure 1.1 A: Foods rich in Calcium

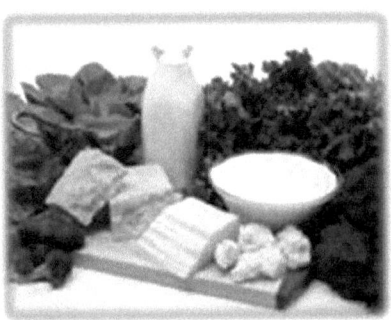

Figure 1.1 B: Foods rich in Vitamin D

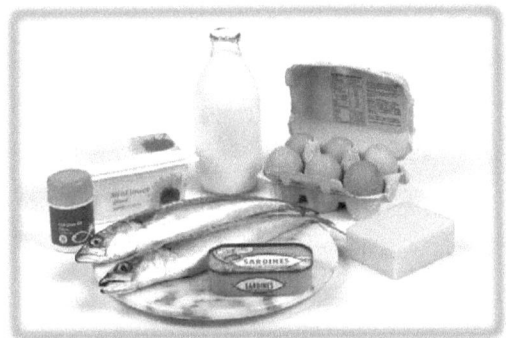

These foods should be included in people's diets in order to avoid calcium and vitamin D deficiency. Calcium rich foods include milk, various cheeses, yoghurts and green leafy vegetables. Vitamin D rich foods include milk, eggs, butter, cheese, cod liver oil, oily fish and sardines as shown above.

(http://www.newrinkles.com/index.php/nutrition/calcium-rich-foods-versus-supplements

http://www.cheapethniceatz.com/2009/11/02/fight-h1n1-with-food/)

1.2 Osteoporosis

The risk factors of developing osteoporosis include being a post-menopausal elderly female, smoking, lack of exercise, being Caucasian and frail due to a poor diet and most likely deficient in calcium and vitamin D. Effective calcium and vitamin D supplementation and weight-bearing exercises can help prevent osteoporosis. However, in certain cases, osteoporosis can begin in utero if the mother is vitamin D deficient. Osteoporosis affects the inorganic component of bone and results in thinning of bone. Consequently, bone loses its strength and so is easily fractured. The typical clinical scenario would be an old lady falling and fracturing her hip and neck of femur. More often than not, patients would be unaware of their bone loss (in post-menopausal women it is about 1% bone loss per year), which is why osteoporosis is referred to as a 'silent' disease. It develops due to a decrease in oestrogen levels in women. However, it also occurs in men due to a decline in bone density as the body ages (Dowd and Stafford, 2008 and Sunyecz J.A., 2008).

In order to minimize risks of developing osteoporosis, it is recommended that exercise, calcium and vitamin D supplementation is taken before the age of 30, as that time would be 'peak bone mass' after which a decline in bone density is observed. Vitamin D deficiency enhances osteoclast proliferation and so increased calcium mobilisation from bone. It is important to note that calcium supplements may interfere with drugs the patient is taking; for instance calcium will increase digoxin to toxicity levels, causing arrhythmia and palpitations. All people above the age of 50 should take a bone density test (dual-energy X-ray absorptiometry implementing the T-score or the Z-score), so as to prevent the risk of bone fractures by starting treatment early on. Pharmacological treatment may be given by using bisphosphonates such as Reclast and Actonel, which act by killing off osteoclasts and effectively inhibiting further bone resorption (Sunyecz J.A., 2008).

Figure 1.2: The progression of osteoporosis after 55 years of age.

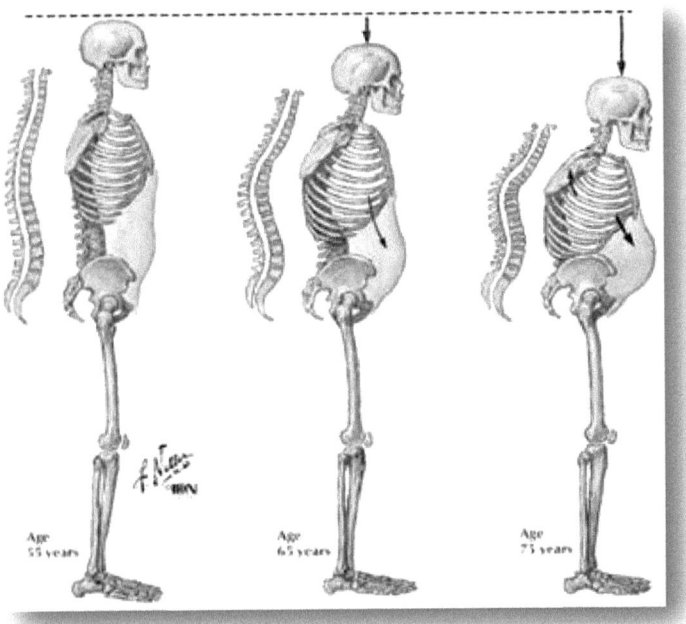

Osteoporosis causes the spaces between one vertebra and the next to decrease, often resulting in compressional fractures. The patient usually suffers from kyphosis and appears shorter in size because of the compressed vertebrae, as shown above.

(http://www.true-beauty-tips.com/osteoporosis-alternatives.html)

Figure 1.3: Cross-section of bone showing increased spaces within trabecular bone and thinning of bone.

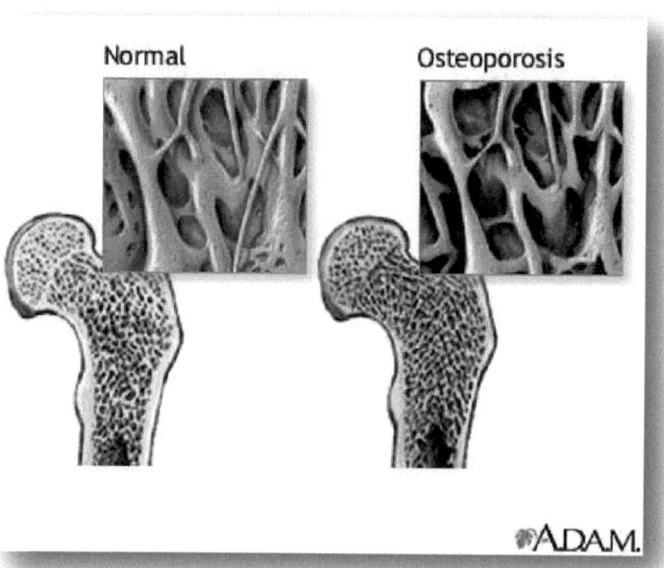

Osteoporosis is a condition in which lack of calcium and vitamin D and age, amongst other factors, induce a higher rate of bone resorption than bone formation. Consequently, the bone matrix is destroyed, cortical bone thins and larger spaces are formed within the bone architecture, as shown above. Bones also appear thinner on X-Rays of osteoporotic patients.

(http://www.chiropractic-help.com/Causes-of-Osteoporosis.html)

1.3   Rickets

This disease manifests in children who are vitamin D deficient and is known as osteomalacia when it occurs in adults, often leading to osteoporosis; which is a decrease of total bone mass, including collagenous tissue in the bone matrix. In the advanced stages, rickets is characterized by growth retardation, epiphysis enlargement in long bones, abnormal projections from the ribcage and bowing or bending of the legs and spine with weak, toneless muscles. This can be reversed by supplementation of high doses vitamin D or calcitriol and ensuring a calcium and phosphate rich diet, to replenish the bone reservoir of ions required for homeostasis (Holick M.F., 2006).

Since vitamin D is deficient in most cases, calcium cannot be absorbed from the intestines to be utilized by bone. The decrease in calcium plasma levels causes an increase in PTH secretion, which in turn enhances RANKL on osteoblasts resulting in increased resorption by osteoclasts. Also, phosphorous reabsorption in inhibited in the kidneys by PTH, causing increased loss of phosphate in the urine. Since serum calcium concentrations are also decreased, there is not enough calcium and phosphorous to ensure laying down of bone by osteoblasts. Also, $1,25\text{-}(OH)_2D_3$ levels are usually normal or high in these children, since excess PTH stimulates its production in the kidneys and so it may appear that the child is not deficient for vitamin D. Coloured peopled were found more likely to be deficient in vitamin D when compared to their white counterparts. Since rickets causes poor mineralization of the whole skeleton, bones which grow rapidly; such as long bones, show the first signs of abnormality especially in infants below 18 months of age (Holick M.F., 2006).

It is essential that people are exposed to enough sunlight as many people are deficient for vitamin D, even though they live in a country with plenty of sunlight. However, this together with an appropriate diet is still not enough for some people because they are genetically 'vitamin D resistant', which leads to rickets. This occurs because a point mutation can occur causing a variation in splicing of VDR; by leaving out exon 8, rendering VDR non-functional (Ma N.S. *et al.*, 2009), or due to a mutation in an enzyme converting $25\text{-}(OH)D_3$ to $1,25\text{-}(OH)_2D_3$. The signs for this condition are aggravated when compared to vitamin D deficiency. The treatment for this condition is pharmacological doses of calcitriol, calcium and phosphorous (Pettifor J.M., 2005).

Figure 1.4: A radiograph showing left femur bowing and an incomplete fracture.

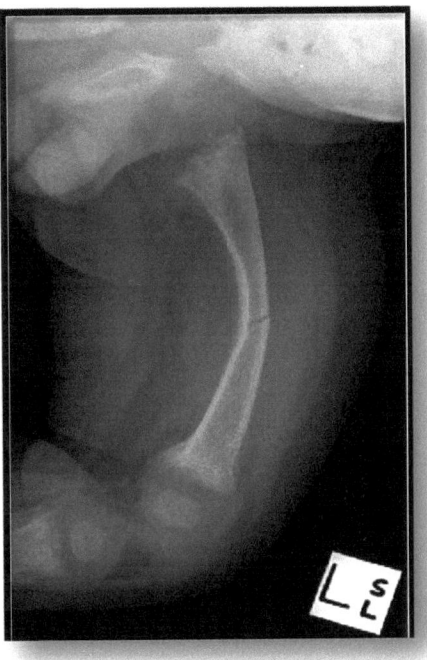

This X-Ray was taken after a 10-month old, coloured boy sustained minor trauma to his left femur. The figure shows bowing of the shaft of femur and an incomplete fracture. He was clearly suffering from vitamin D deficiency either due to a primary cause (inadequate diet and lack of sun exposure) or a secondary cause; such as chronic renal failure, hypophosphataemia, or vitamin-dependent rickets. The bowing and fracture occurred because of lack of calcium in the bones, causing the bones to be weak and unable to support the patient's body. As a result, minor trauma will cause bones to fracture easily since little resistance is offered to stress.

(http://www.radpod.org/2007/01/08/rickets/).

45

Figure 1.5: The clinical signs and symptoms of rickets in a child.

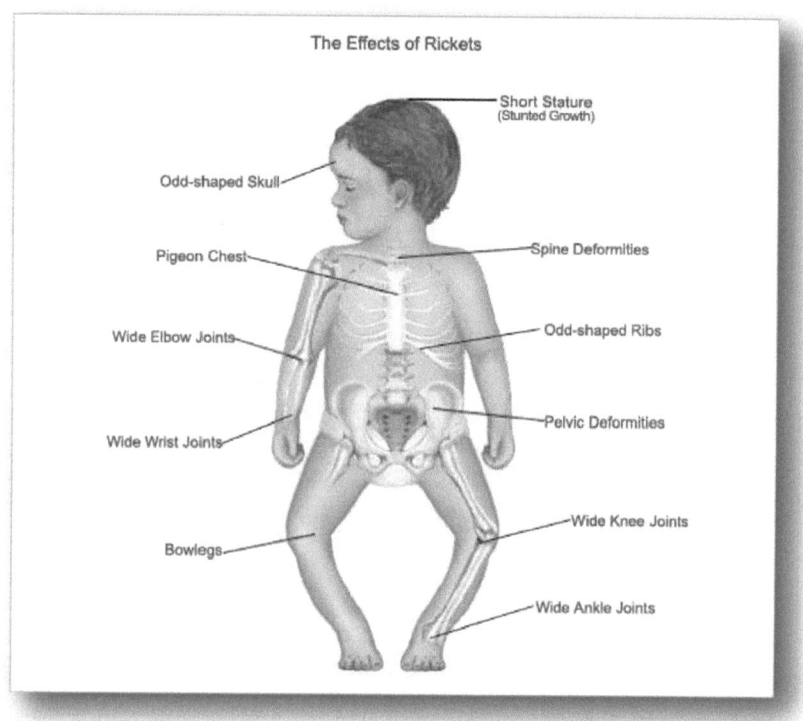

The Effects of Rickets

Short Stature (Stunted Growth)

Odd-shaped Skull

Pigeon Chest

Wide Elbow Joints

Wide Wrist Joints

Bowlegs

Spine Deformities

Odd-shaped Ribs

Pelvic Deformities

Wide Knee Joints

Wide Ankle Joints

The image above shows the classical appearance of a severe case of rickets; including bowed legs, pigeon chest, wide joints, ribs and spinal deformities.

(http://lancastria.net/blog/tag/starvation)

Conclusion

It is remarkable how many people throughout the world are deficient for both vitamin D and calcium without themselves knowing. The best way to reach out to people is by educating the required daily amounts for vitamin D and calcium and showing them the reasons why they are an essential part of our diet, especially in regions of the world lacking sunlight. Research is continually unfolding mysteries of the etiology of major diseases; for instance prostate cancer and colorectal cancer, several of which seeming to involve a deficiency in vitamin D (Dowd and Stafford, 2008). This further stresses the importance of vitamin D and calcium in, not only bone, but our entire body's physiology.

References

1. Douard V., Asgerally A., Sabbagh Y., Sugiura S., Shapses S.A, Casirola D. and Ferrarism R.P. (2010). Dietary Fructose Inhibits Intestinal Calcium Absorption and Induces Vitamin D Insufficiency in CKD. *J. Am. Soc. Nephrol.* 2010 February; **21(2)**: 261–271.

2. Dowd J.E., Stafford D., (2008). The Vitamin D Cure. Wiley J. & Sons, Inc. New Jersey, U.S.A. (ISBN: 978-0-470-56555-1)

3. Holick M.F. (2006). Resurrection of vitamin D deficiency and rickets. American Society for Clinical Investigation. *J. Clin. Invest.* 2006 August; **116(8)**: 2062–2072.

4. Karaplis A.C. (2008). Embryonic Development of Bone and Regulation of Intramembranous and Endochondral Bone Formation. In: Bilezikian J.P., Raisz L.G. and Martin T.J. (Eds.), *Principles of Bone Biology*, Volume 1. (3rd Ed.) (pp. 66-76). Academic Press Inc., New York, U.S.A. (ISBN-13: 978-0123738844)

5. Kumari M., Khazai N.B., Ziegler T.R., Nanes M.S., Abrams S.A. and Tangpricha V. (2010). Vitamin D-mediated calcium absorption in patients with clinically stable Crohn's disease: A pilot study. *Mol. Nutr. Food Res.* 2010 August; **54(8)**: 1085–1091.

6. Ma N.S., Malloy P.J., Pitukcheewanont P., Dreimane D., Geffner M.E. and Feldman D (2009). Hereditary vitamin D resistant rickets: identification of a novel splice site mutation in the vitamin D receptor gene and successful treatment with oral calcium therapy. *Bone.* 2009 October; **45(4)**:743-6.

7. Pettifor, J.M. (2005) Vitamin D deficiency and nutritional rickets in children. In: Feldman D., Pike J.W. and Glorieux F.H. (Eds.). *Vitamin D* (2nd ed.). Elsevier Academic Press, Philadelphia, U.S.A. (ISBN: 0-12-252687-2)

8. Sunyecz J.A. (2008). The use of calcium and vitamin D in the management of osteoporosis. *Ther. Clin. Risk. Manag.* 2008 August; **4(4)**: 827–836. Dove Medical Press Limited.

Websites

- http://lancastria.net/blog/tag/starvation
- http://ods.od.nih.gov/factsheets/calcium
- http://ods.od.nih.gov/factsheets/vitamind
- http://www.cheapethniceatz.com/2009/11/02/fight-h1n1-with-food/
- http://www.chiropractic-help.com/Causes-of-Osteoporosis.html
- http://www.newrinkles.com/index.php/nutrition/calcium-rich-foods-versus-supplements
- http://www.radpod.org/2007/01/08/rickets/
- http://www.true-beauty-tips.com/osteoporosis-alternatives.html

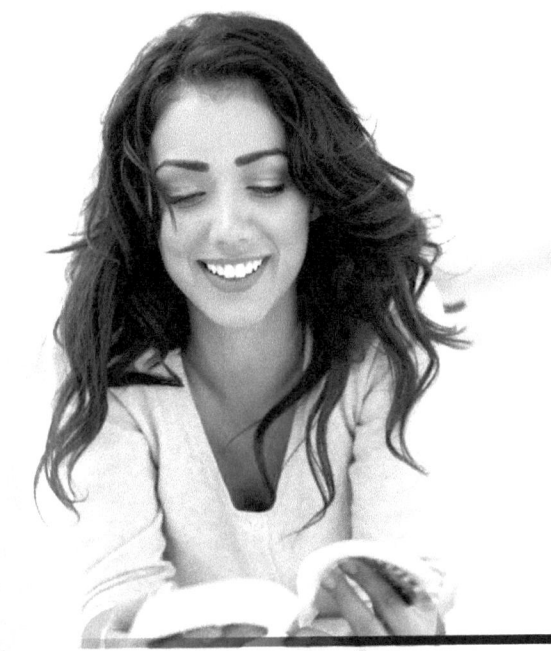
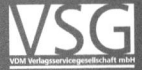

Printed by Books on Demand GmbH, Norderstedt / Germany